ATKINS Ultimate Diet Cookbooks for both Seniors and beginners 2024

Healthy and Effective recipe for weight control and Promoting of long-time wellness

By

Darryl Rojas

Table of contents

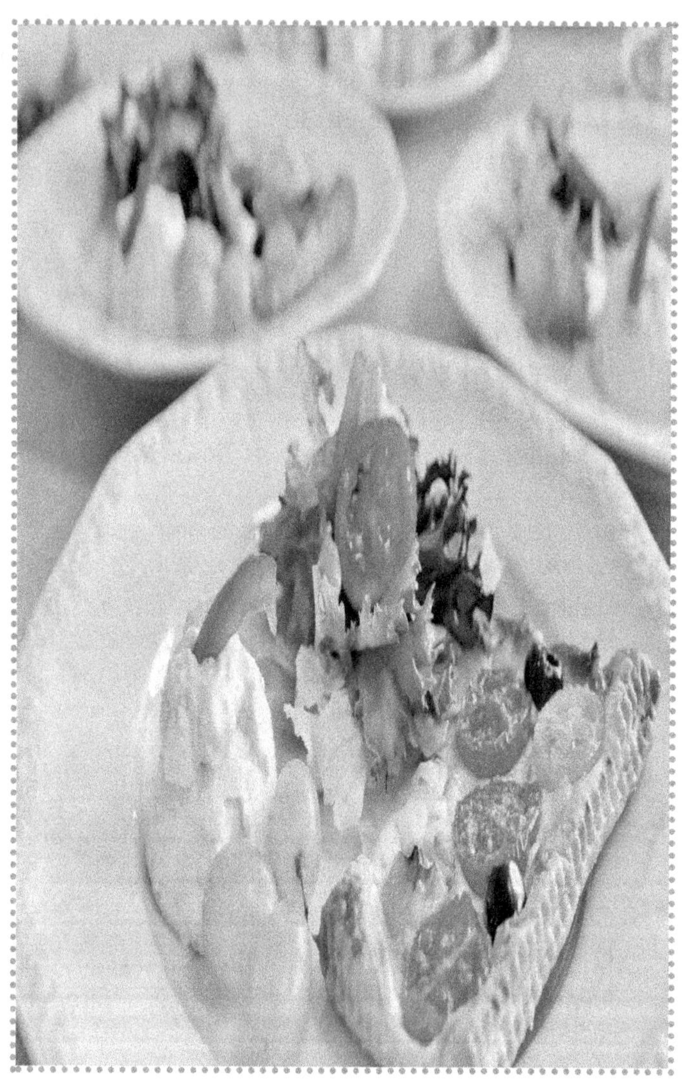

CHAPTER ONE

INTRODUCTION: Embarking on Your Atkins Journey

"The Atkins Adventure: A Journey to Health and Happiness"

Once upon a time, in a world filled with bustling cities and tranquil country sides, there lived a young man named Darryl Rojas. Darryl was like many others in his realm, seeking a path to better health and vitality. He had heard whispers of a miraculous journey called the Atkins diet, a voyage that promised to transform not just bodies, but lives. Intrigued by the tales of success and transformation, Darryl decided to embark on his own Atkins adventure.

With determination burning bright in his heart, Darryl set out on his quest for health and happiness. He gathered his courage, bid farewell to his old habits, and ventured forth into the unknown. Along the way, he encountered challenges and obstacles, but he pressed on, fueled by the promise of a brighter tomorrow.

As Darrly journeyed deeper into the realm of Atkins, he discovered a treasure trove of knowledge and wisdom. He learned the importance of nourishing his body with wholesome foods, rich in protein and healthy fats. He uncovered the secrets of balance, finding harmony in the delicate dance between carbs and nutrients.

Through the ups and downs of his journey, Darryl found strength in the support of his fellow travelers. Together, they shared stories of triumph and setback, lifting each other up with words of encouragement and understanding. In the warmth of their camaraderie, Darryl found solace and inspiration to carry on.

With each passing day, Darrly felt his body grow stronger and his spirit soar higher. He reveled in the newfound energy that coursed through his veins, powering his through each step of his adventure. And as he looked in the mirror, he beheld a reflection of resilience and determination, a testament to the incredible journey she had undertaken.

But Darryl's adventure was not just about physical transformation; it was also a journey of self-discovery and empowerment. Along the way, he unearthed hidden reserves of courage and confidence, realizing that he was capable of far more than he had ever imagined. With each obstacle overcome and each milestone reached,

Darryl grew more assured of his own worth and potential.

And so, dear reader, as you embark on your own Atkins adventure, remember the tale of Darryl Rojas and his journey to health and happiness. Let his story be a beacon of hope and inspiration, guiding you through the challenges and triumphs that lie ahead. For in the world of Atkins, every step you take is a step closer to the best version of yourself.

"Mastering the Atkins Approach: Success Strategies for Both Novices and Seniors"

Embarking on the Atkins journey is a transformative experience, offering a path to improved health and vitality for people of all ages. Whether you're a senior looking to enhance your well-being or a beginner just beginning to explore the world of low-carb living, understanding the Atkins approach is key to achieving lasting success. In this guide, we'll delve into the principles of the Atkins diet, offering in-depth insights and practical tips tailored specifically for seniors and beginners.

Understanding the Atkins Approach:

At the heart of the Atkins approach lies the principle of carbohydrate restriction, which is designed to shift the body's metabolism from relying on carbohydrates for fuel to burning fat instead. By limiting your intake of carbs, you encourage your body to enter a state of ketosis, where it begins to burn stored fat for energy. This metabolic shift not only promotes weight loss but also offers a range of health benefits, including improved blood sugar control, reduced inflammation, and enhanced cognitive function.

The Atkins diet is divided into four phases, each designed to gradually reintroduce carbohydrates into your diet while still promoting weight loss and metabolic health. In the initial phase, known as Phase 1 or the "Induction Phase," carbohydrate intake is limited to 20-25 grams per day, primarily from non-starchy vegetables. This strict phase helps jumpstart ketosis and kickstart weight loss, setting the stage for long-term success.

As you progress through the phases of the Atkins diet, you'll gradually increase your carb intake, incorporating a wider variety of foods while still prioritizing nutrient-dense, whole foods. By the time you reach Phase 4, or the "Maintenance Phase," you'll have established a sustainable way of eating that supports your health and well-being for years to come.

Tips-for-Success:[Seniors Edition

For seniors embarking on the Atkins journey, there are several factors to consider to ensure success and optimize health outcomes. Here are some tips tailored specifically for older adults:

1. **Prioritize Protein**: As we age, maintaining muscle mass becomes increasingly important for overall health and mobility. Make sure to include plenty of high-quality protein sources in your meals, such as lean meats, poultry, fish, eggs, and tofu. Protein not only supports muscle growth and repair but also helps keep you feeling full and satisfied.

2. **Stay Hydrated**: Dehydration can be more common among seniors and can exacerbate certain health conditions. Make it a priority to drink plenty of water throughout the day, aiming for at least 8-10 glasses. You can also include hydrating

foods like cucumber, watermelon, and celery in your diet.

3. **Monitor Electrolytes**: When following a low-carb diet like Atkins, it's important to pay attention to your electrolyte levels, especially sodium, potassium, and magnesium. These minerals play essential roles in hydration, muscle function, and overall health. Include electrolyte-rich foods like leafy greens, avocado, and nuts in your meals, and consider supplementing if needed.

4. **Listen to Your Body**: As you adjust to the Atkins diet, pay close attention to how your body responds to different foods and eating patterns. Seniors may have unique dietary needs and sensitivities, so be mindful of any symptoms or changes in energy levels. Adjust your meal plan accordingly to ensure it meets your individual requirements.

5. **Stay Active**: Regular physical activity is crucial for maintaining muscle mass, mobility, and overall health as we age. Incorporate a variety of exercises into your routine, including strength training, cardio, flexibility, and balance exercises. Find activities that you enjoy and that are appropriate for your fitness level and abilities.

By following these tips and listening to your body's needs, you can navigate the Atkins journey with confidence and achieve your health and wellness goals at any age.

Tips for Success: [Beginners Edition

If you're new to the Atkins diet, getting started can feel overwhelming at first. But with the right guidance and mindset, you can set yourself up for success from the very beginning. Here are some tips to help beginners navigate the Atkins journey:

1. **Educate Yourself**: Take the time to learn about the principles of the Atkins diet and how it works. Familiarize yourself with the different phases, allowable foods, and recommended portion sizes. The more you understand about the program, the better equipped you'll be to make informed choices and stay on track.

2. **Plan Ahead**: Planning is key to staying on course with the Atkins diet, especially in the early stages. Take the time to meal plan and prep, making sure you have plenty of low-carb options on hand for meals and snacks. Stock your kitchen with healthy staples like lean proteins, vegetables, nuts, and seeds to set yourself up for success.

3. **Start Slowly**: Transitioning to a low-carb diet can be a significant change for your body, so it's important to ease into it gradually. Begin by

reducing your carb intake slowly over the course of a few days or weeks, rather than making drastic changes all at once. This can help minimize potential side effects like fatigue or cravings and make the transition more manageable.

4. **Focus on Whole Foods**: While it may be tempting to rely on processed low-carb products, such as bars or shakes, for convenience, try to prioritize whole, nutrient-dense foods whenever possible. Choose fresh vegetables, lean proteins, healthy fats, and low-glycemic fruits to nourish your body and support your health goals.

5. **Stay Flexible**: Remember that the Atkins diet is not one-size-fits-all, and what works for one person may not work for another. Be open to experimenting with different foods and meal plans to find what works best for you. Listen to your body's hunger and fullness cues, and adjust your approach as needed to achieve optimal results.

In brief;
Embarking on the Atkins journey is a powerful step toward improving your health, regardless of your age or level of experience. By understanding the principles of the Atkins approach and implementing practical tips tailored for seniors and beginners, you can navigate the path to success with confidence and ease. Whether you're looking to shed excess weight, improve your metabolic health, or simply feel better in your body, the Atkins diet offers a

roadmap to help you reach your goals and live your best life.

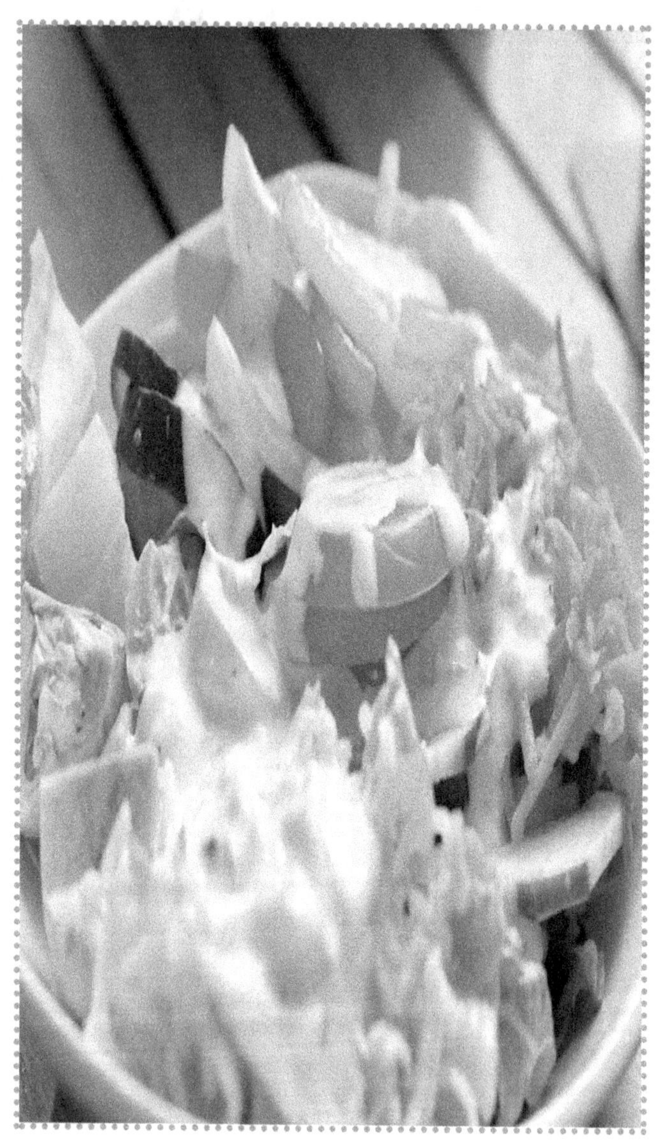

CHAPTER TWO

Culinary Delights for Seniors

In the journey towards improved health and vitality, culinary exploration plays a crucial role, especially for seniors looking to maintain their well-being and savor the joys of food. With the Atkins approach, seniors can enjoy a wide variety of delicious and nutritious meals that cater to their seasoned palates while aligning with their dietary goals. In this guide, we'll explore a collection of senior-friendly starters, soups, stews, appetizers with a twist, and snacks designed to provide sustained energy and satisfaction on the Atkins diet.

Senior-Friendly Starters:

1. **Avocado Shrimp Salad**: Combine diced avocado, cooked shrimp, cherry tomatoes, and cucumbers in a bowl. Dress with a mixture of olive oil, lemon juice, salt, and pepper for a refreshing and protein-packed starter.

2. **Caprese Skewers**: Using fresh mozzarella balls, cherry tomatoes, and basil leaves, thread them onto skewers Drizzle with balsamic glaze and a sprinkle of salt and pepper for a classic Italian-inspired appetizer.

3. **Smoked Salmon Roll-Ups**: Spread cream cheese onto slices of smoked salmon, then roll them up with cucumber slices and avocado. Secure with toothpicks for an elegant and easy-to-eat starter.

Soups and Stews for Seasoned Palates:

1. **Beef and Vegetable Stew**: Slow-cook tender chunks of beef with carrots, celery, onions, and garlic in a rich beef broth. Season with herbs like thyme and rosemary for a comforting and hearty meal that's perfect for chilly evenings.

2. **Creamy Mushroom Soup**: Sauté sliced mushrooms, onions, and garlic in butter until golden brown. Add chicken or vegetable broth and simmer until the flavors meld together. Finish with a splash of heavy cream and a sprinkle of parsley for a velvety, indulgent soup.

3. **Chicken and Spinach Soup**: Simmer chicken breast, spinach, and diced vegetables in chicken broth until the chicken is cooked through and the flavors meld together. Season with salt, pepper, and a touch of lemon juice for a light and nutritious soup option.

Appetizers with a Twist: Low-Carb Delights

1. **Zucchini Fritters**: Grate zucchini and squeeze out excess moisture, then mix with almond flour, eggs, grated cheese, and seasoning. Pan-fry in olive oil until golden brown and crispy for a tasty and low-carb alternative to traditional fritters.

2. **Cauliflower Buffalo Bites**: Toss cauliflower florets in a mixture of buffalo sauce and melted butter, then roast in the oven until tender and caramelized. Serve with a side of ranch dressing for a spicy and satisfying appetizer.

3. **Eggplant Bruschetta**: Slice eggplant into rounds, brush with olive oil, and grill until tender. Top each slice with diced tomatoes, basil, garlic, and a sprinkle of Parmesan cheese for a flavorful twist on classic bruschetta.

Snacks for Sustained Energy:

1. **Almond Butter Celery Sticks**: Spread almond butter on celery sticks and top with a sprinkle of chia seeds for a crunchy and protein-packed snack that's perfect for on-the-go.

2. **Cheese and Pepperoni Roll-Ups**: Roll slices of deli cheese and pepperoni together for a savory and satisfying snack that's high in protein and low in carbs.

3. **Greek Yogurt Parfait**: Layer Greek yogurt with berries, nuts, and a drizzle of honey for a sweet and creamy snack that's packed with protein, fiber, and antioxidants.

In conclusion:

With these senior-friendly starters, soups, stews, appetizers with a twist, and snacks for sustained energy, seniors can indulge in delicious and nutritious meals that support their health and well-being on the Atkins diet. By embracing the principles of low-carb living and incorporating flavorful ingredients and creative twists, seniors can enjoy a diverse and satisfying culinary experience that nourishes both body and soul. So go ahead, explore the possibilities, and savor the delights of Atkins-friendly cuisine with every bite.

CHAPTER THREE

Navigating the Atkins Diet

Embarking on the Atkins diet can be an exciting journey towards improved health and vitality, but for beginners, it can also be overwhelming to navigate the ins and outs of low-carb living. Fear not, as we delve into the beginner's basics, building blocks, essential kitchen tools, techniques, and quick meals tailored to novice cooks on the Atkins diet. By understanding these fundamental aspects, beginners can kickstart their journey with confidence and ease.

Beginner's Basics:

1. **Understanding Carbohydrates**: The cornerstone of the Atkins diet is carbohydrate restriction. Beginners should familiarize themselves with the different types of carbohydrates, including sugars, starches, and fiber, and learn to identify sources of hidden carbs in packaged foods.

2. **Phases of the Atkins Diet**: The Atkins diet is divided into four phases, each with its own set of rules and objectives. Beginners should start with Phase 1, or the "Induction Phase," which restricts carbs to 20-25 grams per day to kickstart ketosis and jumpstart weight loss.

3. **Balancing Macros**: While carbohydrates are limited on the Atkins diet, it's essential to maintain a balance of macronutrients, including protein and fat. Beginners should focus on incorporating lean proteins, healthy fats, and plenty of non-starchy vegetables into their meals to promote satiety and nutritional balance.

Building Blocks of the Atkins Diet:

1. **Protein**: Protein is a critical component of the Atkins diet, as it helps support muscle growth, repair, and satiety. Beginners should include a variety of protein sources in their meals, such as poultry, fish, eggs, tofu, and legumes.

2. **Healthy Fats**: Contrary to popular belief, fats are not the enemy on the Atkins diet; in fact, they're encouraged as a primary source of energy. Beginners should incorporate healthy fats like olive oil, avocados, nuts, and seeds into their meals to promote feelings of fullness and satisfaction.

3. **Non-Starchy Vegetables**: Non-starchy vegetables are low in carbs and high in fiber, making them an essential component of the Atkins diet. Beginners should aim to fill their plates with a colorful array of veggies like leafy greens, peppers,

broccoli, and cauliflower to boost nutrient intake and promote digestive health.

Essential Kitchen Tools and Techniques:

1. **Food Scale**: A food scale is an invaluable tool for beginners on the Atkins diet, allowing them to accurately measure portion sizes and track their carbohydrate intake. Investing in a digital food scale can help ensure consistency and accuracy in meal planning and preparation.

2. **Vegetable Spiralizer**: A vegetable spiralizer is a fun and versatile tool that allows beginners to transform vegetables like zucchini, carrots, and sweet potatoes into low-carb alternatives to pasta and noodles. Spiralized veggies can add texture and flavor to dishes while keeping carb counts low.

3. **Cast Iron Skillet**: A cast iron skillet is a kitchen staple that's perfect for cooking protein-rich foods like steak, chicken, and fish. Beginners should season their skillet properly and learn how to cook with it to achieve delicious and evenly cooked meals every time.

Quick and Easy Meals for Novice Cooks:

1. **Grilled Chicken Caesar Salad**: Season chicken breasts with herbs and spices, then grill until cooked through. Serve sliced chicken over a bed of romaine lettuce, cherry tomatoes, and shaved Parmesan cheese, dressed with Caesar dressing for a quick and satisfying meal.

2. **Egg Roll in a Bowl**: Brown ground turkey or pork in a skillet with garlic, ginger, and soy sauce. Add shredded cabbage, carrots, and onions, and cook until vegetables are tender. Serve topped with green onions and sesame seeds for a low-carb twist on a classic egg roll.

3. **Cauliflower Fried Rice**: Using a food processor, pulse the cauliflower florets until they resemble rice grains.. Sauté with diced vegetables, scrambled eggs, and soy sauce until heated through. Garnish with chopped green onions and sesame seeds for a flavorful and satisfying dish.

Conclusion:
With these beginner's basics, building blocks, essential kitchen tools, techniques, and quick meals, novice cooks can embark on their Atkins journey with confidence and ease. By understanding the principles of low-carb living, mastering essential cooking skills, and

incorporating flavorful ingredients and creative recipes, beginners can enjoy a diverse and satisfying culinary experience while achieving their health and wellness goals. So don't hesitate to dive in, explore the possibilities, and savor the delights of Atkins-friendly cuisine with every bite.

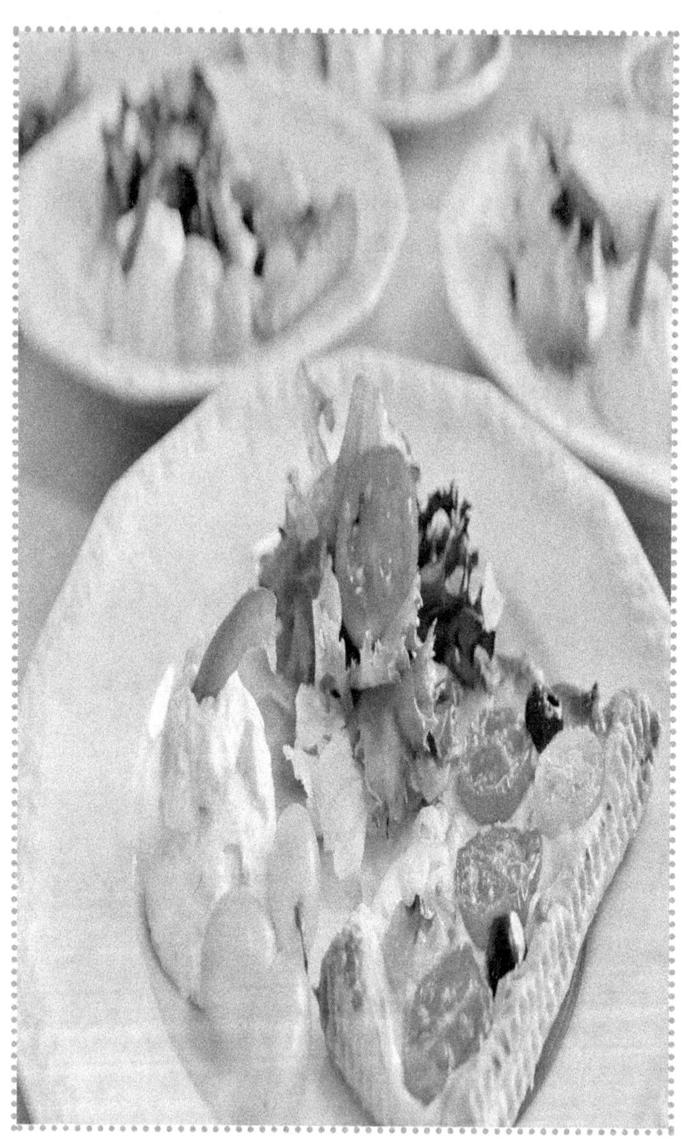

CHAPTER FOUR

Salad Sensations

Salads are not just a meal; they're a canvas for culinary creativity, offering endless possibilities for fresh flavors, vibrant colors, and nourishing ingredients. For those following the Atkins diet, salads can be a delicious and satisfying way to enjoy a wide variety of nutrient-dense foods while keeping carb counts low. In this guide, we'll explore a collection of salad sensations, featuring fresh and flavorful creations, dressings, toppings, and a complete nutritional guide tailored for Atkins followers.

Fresh and Flavorful Salad Creations:

1. **Mediterranean Greek Salad**: Toss together chopped romaine lettuce, cherry tomatoes, cucumber slices, red onion, Kalamata olives, and crumbled feta cheese in a bowl. Dress with a mixture of olive oil, lemon juice, garlic, and oregano for a taste of the Mediterranean.

2. **Asian-Inspired Chicken Salad**: Top mixed greens with shredded rotisserie chicken, shredded carrots, sliced bell peppers, edamame, and sliced

almonds. Drizzle with a homemade sesame ginger dressing made with soy sauce, sesame oil, rice vinegar, and ginger for an Asian-inspired twist.

3. Southwestern Steak Salad: Grill thinly sliced steak seasoned with chili powder, cumin, and garlic until cooked to your desired doneness. Serve over a bed of mixed greens with black beans, corn, avocado slices, diced tomatoes, and shredded cheese. Finish with a dollop of salsa and a squeeze of lime for a taste of the Southwest.

Dressings and Toppings for Every Taste:

1. **Creamy Avocado Dressing**: Blend ripe avocado with Greek yogurt, lime juice, garlic, cilantro, and a splash of water until smooth and creamy. This dressing adds richness and flavor to any salad while keeping carb counts low.

2. **Balsamic Vinaigrette**: Whisk together balsamic vinegar, Dijon mustard, minced garlic, honey (optional), and olive oil until emulsified. Season with salt and pepper to taste for a tangy and versatile dressing that pairs well with a variety of salads.

3. **Toppings Galore**: Get creative with toppings to add texture and flavor to your salads. Try toasted nuts and seeds, crumbled cheese, crispy bacon bits, hard-boiled eggs, roasted vegetables, fresh herbs, and sliced avocado for endless variety and enjoyment.

Salad Meals: A Complete Nutritional Guide

1. **Protein**: Incorporating protein into your salads is essential for satiety and muscle maintenance. Include sources like grilled chicken, shrimp, salmon, tofu, hard-boiled eggs, or beans to add substance and nutrition to your meal.

2. **Fats**: Healthy fats are a cornerstone of the Atkins diet and can be easily incorporated into salads through ingredients like avocado, olive oil, nuts, seeds, and cheese. These fats not only add flavor and richness but also help keep you feeling full and satisfied.

3. **Carbohydrates**: While the Atkins diet restricts overall carb intake, non-starchy vegetables like leafy greens, cucumbers, bell peppers, and tomatoes are encouraged in abundance. These veggies provide essential vitamins, minerals, and fiber without spiking blood sugar levels.

4. **Fiber**: Fiber is important for digestive health and can be found in abundance in vegetables, nuts, seeds, and low-carb fruits like berries. Including fiber-rich ingredients in your salads helps promote fullness and supports overall gut health.

5. **Portion Control**: While salads can be a nutritious choice on the Atkins diet, it's important to practice portion control to ensure you're not overeating. Pay attention to serving sizes of protein, fats, and carbohydrates, and aim to fill your plate with a balance of nutrient-dense foods.

In Conclusion:
With these salad sensations, featuring fresh and flavorful creations, dressings, toppings, and a complete nutritional guide tailored for Atkins followers, you can enjoy delicious and satisfying meals while staying on track with your health and wellness goals. By incorporating a variety of ingredients, flavors, and textures into your salads, you can create nourishing and delicious meals that nourish your body and delight your taste buds. So go ahead, explore the possibilities, and savor the joys of salad sensations on the Atkins diet.

CHAPTER FIVE

"Main Course Magic: Protein-Packed Plates for Seniors on the Atkins Diet"

As we age, maintaining muscle mass, supporting bone health, and managing weight become increasingly important for overall well-being. Protein-packed main courses play a crucial role in meeting these needs while satisfying the palate and providing essential nutrients. For seniors following the Atkins diet, which emphasizes low-carb, high-protein meals, mastering main course magic is key to achieving health and vitality. In this guide, we'll explore a variety of protein-packed plates tailored for seniors on the Atkins diet, along with a beginner's guide to cooking with confidence and a collection of one-pot wonders and easy entrees to simplify mealtime.

Main-Course-Magic: Protein-Packed-Plates-for Seniors on Atkins

1. **Grilled Salmon with Lemon-Herb Butter**: Marinate salmon fillets in a mixture of olive oil, lemon juice, garlic, and fresh herbs such as dill or parsley. Grill until cooked through and flaky, then top with a dollop of lemon-herb butter for a flavorful and nutritious main course rich in omega-3 fatty acids.

2. **Balsamic Glazed Chicken Thighs**: Season chicken thighs with salt, pepper, and dried herbs, then sear in a skillet until golden brown. Drizzle with a reduction of balsamic vinegar and honey (optional) and simmer until the sauce thickens and coats the chicken. Serve with roasted vegetables for a satisfying low-carb meal.

3. **Beef and Broccoli Stir-Fry**: Sauté thinly sliced beef sirloin with garlic, ginger, and sliced bell peppers in a wok or skillet until browned. Add broccoli florets and a splash of soy sauce, then stir-fry until the broccoli is tender-crisp. Serve over cauliflower rice for a delicious and filling Asian-inspired dish.

Beginner's Guide to Cooking with Confidence:

1. **Start Simple**: Begin your culinary journey with simple recipes that require minimal ingredients and basic cooking techniques. Focus on mastering the fundamentals, such as sautéing, grilling, and roasting, before moving on to more complex dishes.

2. **Build Your Skills**: As you gain confidence in the kitchen, gradually expand your repertoire by trying new ingredients and experimenting with different flavors and cuisines. Don't be afraid to make mistakes; learning from them is part of the journey to becoming a confident cook.

3. **Embrace Adaptability**: Flexibility is key to successful cooking, especially when following a specific dietary plan like Atkins. Learn to adapt recipes to suit your tastes and nutritional needs, substituting ingredients as necessary and experimenting with flavor combinations to create meals that you truly enjoy.

One-Pot Wonders and Easy Entrees:

1. **Spaghetti Squash Carbonara**: Roast spaghetti squash halves until tender, then use a fork to shred the flesh into "noodles." Toss with cooked bacon or pancetta, beaten eggs, grated Parmesan cheese, and chopped parsley for a low-carb twist on classic carbonara.

2. **Lemon Garlic Shrimp and Zoodles**: Sauté shrimp in garlic-infused olive oil until pink and opaque, then toss with spiralized zucchini (zoodles), lemon zest, and red pepper flakes. Serve with a sprinkle of grated Parmesan cheese for a light and refreshing meal that comes together in minutes.

3. **Turkey and Vegetable Skillet**: Brown ground turkey in a skillet with diced onions, bell peppers, and zucchini until cooked through. Season with taco seasoning or your favorite herbs and spices, then serve with shredded lettuce, diced tomatoes, avocado slices, and a dollop of Greek yogurt for a quick and satisfying Tex-Mex-inspired dinner.

In Conclusion:
With these protein-packed plates, beginner's guide to cooking with confidence, and one-pot wonders and easy entrees tailored for seniors on the Atkins diet, mealtime becomes an opportunity to nourish the body and delight the senses. By embracing simple yet flavorful recipes, building culinary skills with patience and practice, and exploring the versatility of one-pot meals, seniors can enjoy delicious and nutritious main courses that support their health and well-being. So fire up the stove, sharpen your knives, and embark on a journey of main course magic with Atkins as your guide.

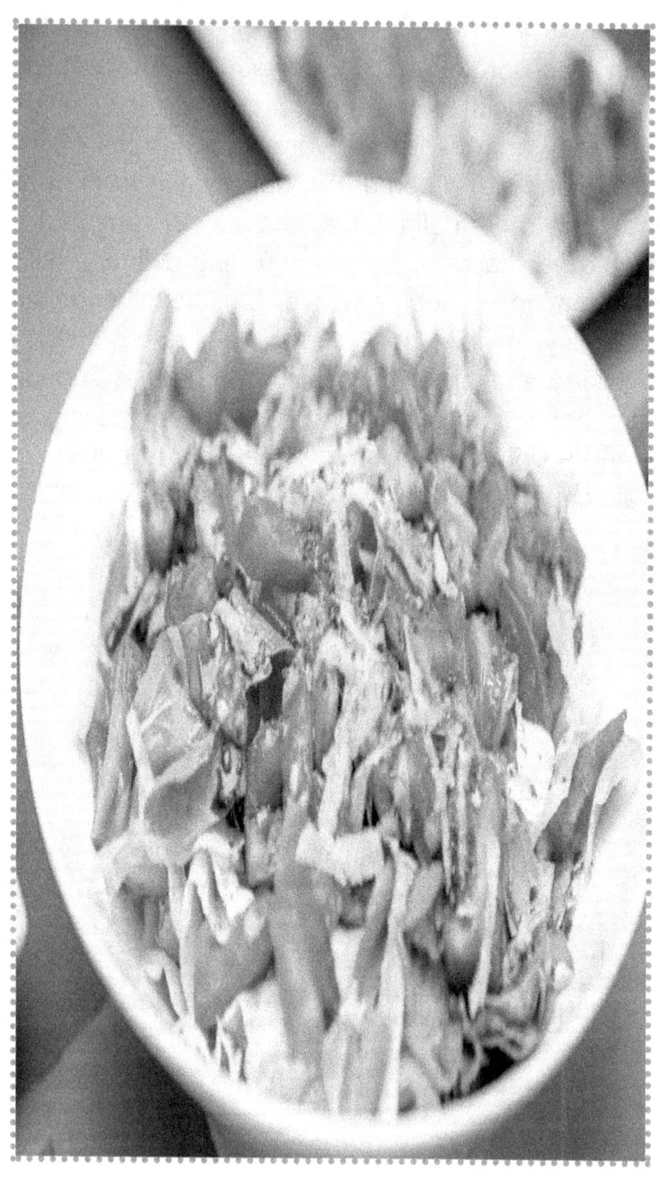

CHAPTER SIX

"Sides and Sips: Elevating Your Atkins Experience"

No meal is complete without the perfect accompaniments to complement the main course and tantalize the taste buds. For those following the Atkins diet, sides and sips play a crucial role in creating a well-rounded and satisfying dining experience. From vegetable varieties that serve as side dish solutions to flavorful beverages beyond water and low-carb cocktails and mocktails for every occasion, there's a world of culinary delights waiting to be explored. In this guide, we'll delve into the realm of sides and sips, offering a plethora of options to elevate your Atkins experience.

Vegetable Varieties: [Side Dish Solutions]

1. **Roasted Brussels Sprouts with Bacon**: Toss halved Brussels sprouts with olive oil, salt, and pepper, then roast in the oven until caramelized and tender. Finish with crispy bacon bits for a savory and satisfying side dish that pairs perfectly with any protein.

2. **Garlic Parmesan Zucchini Noodles**: Sauté spiralized zucchini noodles (zoodles) in garlic-infused olive oil until tender-crisp, then toss with grated Parmesan cheese, chopped parsley, salt, and pepper. This low-carb alternative to pasta is both flavorful and nutritious.

3. **Cauliflower Mash**: Steam or boil cauliflower florets until soft, then mash with a potato masher or blend until smooth. Stir in butter, cream, garlic powder, and salt to taste for a creamy and indulgent side dish that's perfect for replacing mashed potatoes.

Beverages Beyond Water: Flavorful Hydration:

1. **Infused Water**: Elevate your hydration game by infusing water with fresh fruits, herbs, and spices. Try combinations like cucumber and mint, lemon and basil, or strawberries and rosemary for a refreshing and flavorful alternative to plain water.

2. **Iced Herbal Tea**: Brew herbal teas like peppermint, chamomile, or hibiscus, then chill in the refrigerator and serve over ice for a caffeine-free and hydrating beverage option. Sweeten with a splash of liquid stevia if desired.

3. **Sparkling Water with Citrus**: Add a splash of citrus flavor to sparkling water by squeezing in fresh lemon, lime, or orange juice. Garnish with a twist of citrus peel for an elegant and refreshing drink that's perfect for any occasion.

Low-Carb-Cocktails,and Mocktails for Every Occasion:

1. **Vodka Soda with Lime**: Mix vodka with soda water and a squeeze of fresh lime juice for a classic low-carb cocktail that's light and refreshing. Garnish with a lime wedge for a pop of color and flavor.

2. **Mojito Mocktail**: Muddle fresh mint leaves with lime juice and a splash of liquid stevia in a glass. Top with soda water and crushed ice for a refreshing and alcohol-free twist on the classic mojito.

3. **Skinny Margarita**: Shake tequila, fresh lime juice, and a splash of orange liqueur (optional) with ice in a cocktail shaker. Strain into a salt-rimmed glass filled with ice for a tangy and low-carb version of this beloved cocktail.

-With these sides and sips, ranging from vegetable varieties to flavorful beverages beyond water and low-carb cocktails and mocktails, the Atkins dining experience becomes a journey of culinary exploration and delight. By incorporating a variety of ingredients, flavors, and textures into your meals and beverages, you can create a truly satisfying and enjoyable dining experience that supports your health and wellness goals. So raise a glass, savor the flavors, and let sides and sips take your Atkins experience to new heights.

CHAPTER SEVEN

"Indulging in Desserts for Wellness: Sweet Treats Without the Guilt"

Desserts hold a special place in the culinary world, offering a moment of indulgence and satisfaction at the end of a meal. For those following the Atkins diet, desserts can still be enjoyed while supporting health and wellness goals. By choosing ingredients carefully and finding creative ways to satisfy the sweet tooth without derailing progress, dessert time becomes an opportunity to indulge without guilt. In this guide, we'll explore a variety of desserts for wellness on Atkins, featuring sweet treats without the guilt, senior-friendly sweets in moderation, and beginner's baking for simple confections.

Desserts for Wellness:

1. **Avocado Chocolate Mousse**: Blend ripe avocados with unsweetened cocoa powder, a splash of almond milk, and a touch of vanilla extract until smooth and creamy. Sweeten with a low-carb sweetener like erythritol or stevia, then chill until set for a rich and indulgent dessert that's packed with healthy fats.

2. **Berry Parfait**: Layer mixed berries with Greek yogurt or whipped cream sweetened with stevia in a glass or jar for a colorful and refreshing dessert option. Top with a sprinkle of chopped nuts or shredded coconut for added crunch and texture.

3. **Peanut Butter Protein Balls**: Mix together peanut butter, protein powder, coconut flour, and a drizzle of sugar-free syrup until well combined. Roll into bite-sized balls and chill until firm for a protein-packed treat that's perfect for satisfying cravings on the go.

Sweet Treats Without the Guilt:

1. **Coconut Flour Pancakes**: Combine coconut flour, eggs, almond milk, and a pinch of baking powder to make a thick batter. Cook in a skillet until golden brown, then serve with a dollop of Greek yogurt and fresh berries for a satisfying breakfast or dessert option.

2. **Chia Seed Pudding**: Mix chia seeds with unsweetened almond milk, vanilla extract, and a sprinkle of cinnamon in a jar or bowl. Let sit in the refrigerator overnight to thicken, then top with sliced fruit and a drizzle of sugar-free syrup for a creamy and nutritious pudding.

3. **Dark Chocolate Covered Almonds**: Melt sugar-free dark chocolate in a double boiler, then dip whole almonds into the chocolate until coated. Place on a parchment-lined baking sheet and chill until set for a crunchy and satisfying snack that satisfies the sweet tooth without derailing progress.

Senior-Friendly-Sweets: [Indulgence in Moderation]

1. **Baked Apples with Cinnamon**: Core apples and sprinkle with cinnamon and a touch of sweetener, then bake until tender for a warm and comforting dessert that's reminiscent of apple pie without the crust.

2. **Sugar-Free Cheesecake Bites**: Make a simple cheesecake filling using cream cheese, Greek yogurt, eggs, and vanilla extract sweetened with erythritol or stevia. Pour into mini muffin tins and bake until set, then chill until firm for a creamy and decadent treat.

3. **Frozen Yogurt Bark**: Spread Greek yogurt sweetened with stevia onto a parchment-lined baking sheet, then top with sliced fruit, nuts, and a drizzle of sugar-free syrup. Freeze until solid, then break into pieces for a refreshing and customizable dessert option.

Beginner's Baking: [Simple Confections]

1. **Almond Flour Cookies**: Mix together almond flour, butter, eggs, and a low-carb sweetener like erythritol or stevia until a dough forms. Shape into cookies and bake until golden brown for a chewy and satisfying treat.

2. **Coconut Flour Brownies**: Combine coconut flour, cocoa powder, eggs, coconut oil, and a pinch of baking powder in a bowl until well combined. Pour into a baking dish and bake until set, then let cool before slicing into squares for a rich and fudgy dessert.

3. **Lemon Poppy Seed Muffins**: Whisk together almond flour, coconut flour, eggs, lemon zest, poppy seeds, and a low-carb sweetener until smooth. Divide into muffin cups and bake until golden brown for a citrusy and delightful baked treat.

CHAPTER EIGHT

Navigating Nutrition with Atkins:

Atkins is a well-known dietary approach that emphasizes low-carbohydrate intake to promote weight loss and overall health. Understanding the principles of Atkins involves grasping not only the macronutrient composition but also the significance of micronutrients and how they align with specific nutritional needs, particularly for seniors. Additionally, mastering the art of reading labels and making informed choices is essential for success on the Atkins journey. Let's examine each in more detail.

Understanding Macronutrients:

Macronutrients, namely carbohydrates, proteins, and fats, play pivotal roles in the Atkins diet. The foundation of Atkins lies in controlling carbohydrate intake, particularly those with high glycemic indices, to stabilize blood sugar levels and trigger the body's fat-burning mode. This entails consuming primarily low-carb vegetables, lean proteins, and healthy fats. Proteins are essential for muscle repair and growth, while fats provide sustained energy and support various bodily functions.

In Atkins, the focus is on "net carbs," which subtracts fiber and sugar alcohols from total carbohydrates, as these components have minimal impact on blood sugar levels. By monitoring net carbs, followers can sustain ketosis, a metabolic state where the body burns fat for fuel efficiently. While carbohydrates are limited, adequate protein intake is encouraged to prevent muscle loss and promote satiety. Healthy fats, such as those from avocados, nuts, and olive oil, are emphasized for their role in heart health and overall well-being.

Understanding Micronutrients:

While the Atkins diet primarily emphasizes macronutrients, the importance of micronutrients should not be overlooked. Micronutrients, including vitamins and minerals, are essential for various physiological processes, such as metabolism, immune function, and bone health. Since certain food groups may be restricted or limited on the Atkins diet, ensuring adequate micronutrient intake is crucial for overall health and vitality.

To optimize micronutrient intake on Atkins, focus on consuming a variety of nutrient-dense foods. Incorporate colorful vegetables like spinach, broccoli, and bell peppers, which are rich in vitamins A, C, and K, as well as minerals like potassium and magnesium. Additionally, include sources of healthy fats such as fatty fish (salmon, mackerel), which provide omega-3 fatty acids vital for heart health and cognitive function.

Senior-Specific-Nutritional Needs;

Seniors have unique nutritional needs due to factors such as age-related changes in metabolism, muscle mass, and nutrient absorption. While the principles of Atkins can be beneficial for older adults seeking weight management and improved health, modifications may be necessary to address senior-specific concerns.

One consideration for seniors on Atkins is ensuring an adequate intake of protein to support muscle maintenance and prevent age-related sarcopenia (muscle loss). Including protein-rich foods such as eggs, poultry, and Greek yogurt can help meet protein needs without exceeding carbohydrate limits. Additionally, seniors may benefit from focusing on nutrient-dense foods that provide essential vitamins and minerals to support overall health and vitality.

Another aspect to consider is hydration, as older adults may have decreased thirst sensation and be at higher risk of dehydration. Encouraging adequate fluid intake, primarily from water and herbal teas, is essential for maintaining hydration and supporting metabolic processes.

Beginner's Guide to Reading Labels and Making Choices;

Successfully navigating the grocery aisles while following the Atkins diet requires mastering the art of reading labels and making informed choices. By understanding how to interpret nutrition labels, you can identify foods that align with your dietary goals and avoid hidden sources of carbohydrates.

When reading labels on Atkins, focus on the total carbohydrate content per serving, paying attention to both sugars and fiber. Subtracting fiber from total carbs gives you the net carb count, which is what matters most in the Atkins approach. Look for foods with lower net carbs and prioritize whole, unprocessed options whenever possible.

In addition to carbohydrates, pay attention to the ingredient list to identify any hidden sugars or additives that may hinder your progress on Atkins. Ingredients like high-fructose corn syrup, maltodextrin, and hydrogenated oils should be avoided, as they can spike blood sugar levels and derail ketosis.

Furthermore, be mindful of portion sizes and serving recommendations, as these can vary among products. Opt for single-ingredient foods and minimally processed options to ensure you're fueling your body with quality nutrients while staying within your carbohydrate limits.

In conclusion, mastering nutrition on Atkins involves understanding the roles of macronutrients and micronutrients, tailoring the diet to meet senior-specific needs, and becoming adept at reading labels and making informed choices. By embracing these principles, you can embark on a successful Atkins journey that supports your health, vitality, and weight management goals.

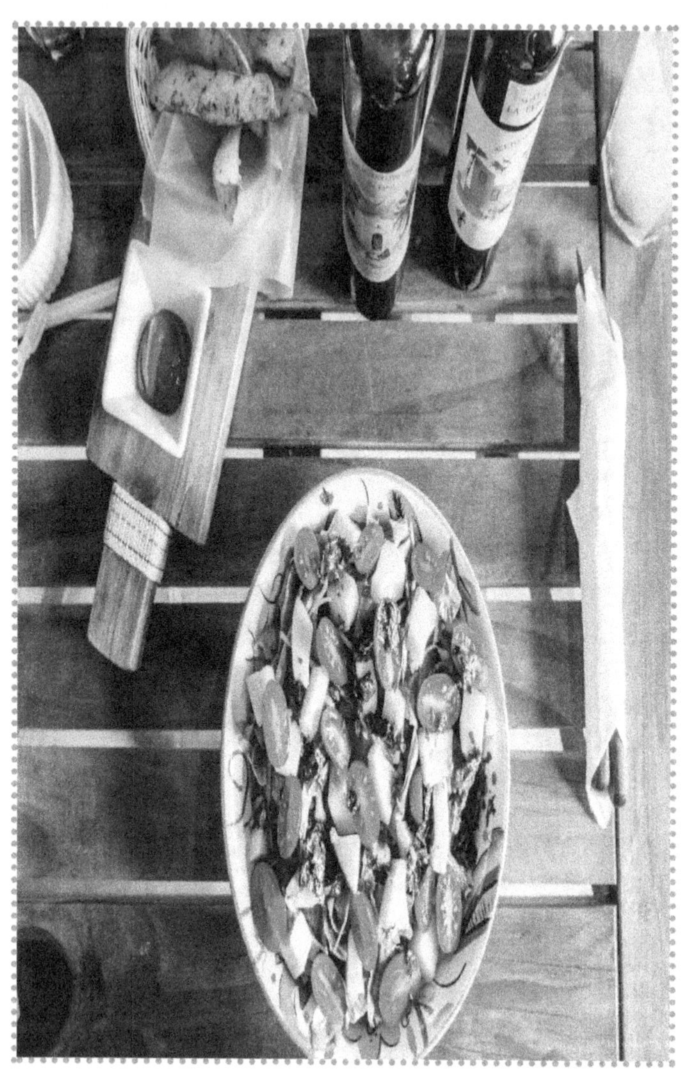

CHAPTER NINE

Meal Planning Made Easy:

Meal planning is a cornerstone of success on the Atkins diet, providing structure and ensuring that you have nourishing, low-carb options readily available. Whether you're a seasoned Atkins follower or just starting out, mastering the art of meal planning can simplify your journey to better health and weight management.

Start by taking inventory of your pantry, refrigerator, and freezer to see what low-carb staples you already have on hand. This will help you build your shopping list and minimize food waste. Next, brainstorm a list of your favorite Atkins-friendly meals and snacks, taking into account your dietary preferences and any specific nutritional goals you have in mind.

Once you have your list, schedule a dedicated time each week to plan your meals and snacks for the upcoming days. This could involve browsing Atkins-approved recipes online, flipping through cookbooks, or simply jotting down ideas based on your favorite ingredients. Consider batch cooking large quantities of protein, vegetables, and grains to streamline meal prep and save time during the week.

As you plan your meals, aim for a balance of protein, healthy fats, and fiber-rich carbohydrates from non-starchy vegetables. Experiment with different flavor profiles and cooking methods to keep things interesting and prevent mealtime boredom. And don't forget to include plenty of hydration in your plan, whether it's through water, herbal tea, or low-carb beverages.

By investing a little time and effort into meal planning each week, you can set yourself up for success on the Atkins diet and make healthy eating a breeze.

Weekly Menu Ideas for Seniors:

Planning a week's worth of meals on the Atkins diet can be both simple and delicious, even for seniors looking to prioritize their health and well-being. Here's a sample menu to inspire your weekly meal planning:

Monday:

- Breakfast: Scrambled eggs with spinach and mushrooms cooked in olive oil.
- Lunch consists of grilled chicken salad topped with avocado, cucumber, cherry tomatoes, and mixed greens.
- Dinner: Baked salmon with roasted asparagus and cauliflower rice.

Tuesday:

- Breakfast: Greek yogurt topped with berries and a sprinkle of nuts.
- Lunch: Turkey and cheese roll-ups with lettuce wraps and sliced bell peppers.
- Dinner: Zucchini noodles with marinara sauce and grilled shrimp.

Wednesday:

- Breakfast: Veggie omelet made with bell peppers, onions, and cheese.
- Lunch: Tuna salad stuffed in cucumber boats with a side of baby carrots.
- Dinner: Beef stir-fry with broccoli, snap peas, and sesame ginger sauce.

Thursday:

- Cottage cheese with sliced peaches and honey drizzled over it for breakfast.
- Lunch: Egg salad lettuce wraps with sliced avocado and cherry tomatoes.
-Supper consists of roasted Brussels sprouts, baked chicken thighs, and a side salad.

Friday:

- Breakfast: Smoked salmon and cream cheese on a low-carb wrap.
- Lunch: Cobb salad with grilled chicken, bacon, hard-boiled eggs, and avocado.

- Dinner: Cauliflower crust pizza topped with marinara, mozzarella, and your favorite veggies.

Saturday:

- Breakfast: Almond flour pancakes with sugar-free syrup and a side of bacon.
- Lunch: Shrimp and avocado salad with mixed greens, cherry tomatoes, and cucumbers.
- Dinner: Grilled steak with sautéed spinach and mashed cauliflower.

Sunday:

- Breakfast: Crustless quiche with spinach, mushrooms, and feta cheese.
- Lunch: Chicken Caesar salad with romaine lettuce, grilled chicken, parmesan cheese, and Caesar dressing.
- Dinner: Baked cod with roasted asparagus and spaghetti squash.

Feel free to customize these menu ideas based on your personal preferences and dietary needs. Always stay hydrated and pay attention to your body's signals of hunger and fullness throughout the day.

Beginner's Batch Cooking: -> Time-Saving Tips:

Batch cooking is a game-changer for anyone following the Atkins diet, especially beginners looking to streamline meal prep and save time during busy weekdays. By preparing large quantities of Atkins-friendly recipes ahead of time, you can ensure that you always have nutritious options on hand and avoid the temptation of reaching for less healthy convenience foods.

Here are some time-saving tips to help you master batch cooking on Atkins:

1. **Plan Your Menu**: Start by selecting a few Atkins-approved recipes that you enjoy and that can easily be scaled up to make larger batches. Choose recipes that incorporate a variety of proteins, vegetables, and healthy fats to keep your meals balanced and satisfying.

2. **Invest in Storage Containers**: Stock up on high-quality storage containers in various sizes to store your batch-cooked meals and snacks. Opt for containers that are freezer-safe, microwave-safe, and easy to stack for efficient storage.

3. **Prep Your Ingredients**: Before you start cooking, take the time to chop, slice, and prep your ingredients so that everything is ready to go when it's time to cook. This will help streamline the cooking process and make assembly a breeze.

4. **Cook in Bulk**: Once you're ready to start cooking, double or triple the quantities of your chosen recipes to make larger batches. Use large pots, pans, and baking sheets to accommodate the increased volume.

5. **Embrace One-Pot Meals**: Look for recipes that can be cooked in a single pot or pan to minimize cleanup and simplify the cooking process. Soups, stews, and casseroles are excellent options for batch cooking and can easily be portioned out for future meals.

6. **Use Your Freezer**: Don't be afraid to freeze batch-cooked meals and snacks for later use. Divide larger batches into individual portions and freeze them in labeled containers or freezer bags for easy grab-and-go convenience.

7. **Rotate Your Stock**: To prevent food waste and keep your meals exciting, rotate your batch-cooked items regularly. Aim to consume frozen meals within a few weeks and replenish your stash with fresh batches as needed.

By incorporating batch cooking into your Atkins routine, you can save time, reduce stress, and set yourself up for success on your low-carb journey.

Eating Out on Atkins: [Seniors and Beginners Edition:

Eating out while following the Atkins diet can present unique challenges, especially for seniors and beginners who may be navigating unfamiliar menus and social situations. However, with a little preparation and know-how, you can enjoy dining out while staying true to your low-carb lifestyle.

Here are some tips for dining out on Atkins, tailored specifically for seniors and beginners:

1. **Do Your Research**: Before heading to a restaurant, take some time to review the menu online and look for low-carb options. Many restaurants now offer nutritional information on their websites, making it easier to plan ahead and make informed choices.

2. **Choose Protein-Rich Options**: When dining out on Atkins, prioritize protein-rich dishes such as grilled chicken, fish, steak, or tofu. These options will help keep you feeling satisfied and provide essential nutrients to support muscle health and satiety.

3. **Skip the Bread Basket**: To avoid temptation, politely decline the bread basket or any complimentary chips or crackers offered at the beginning of the meal. Instead, focus on enjoying a protein-rich appetizer or salad to kick off your dining experience.

4. **Opt for Low-Carb Sides**: Many restaurants offer a variety of side dishes that can easily be modified to fit your low-carb needs. Instead of traditional starches like rice, potatoes, or pasta, consider substituting with steamed vegetables, side salads, or sautéed greens.

5. **Be Mindful of Sauces and Dressings**: Pay attention to sauces, dressings.

CHAPTER TEN

CONCLUSION

Continuing Your Atkins Journey:

Embarking on the Atkins diet is just the beginning of your journey to improved health, vitality, and weight management. As you continue on your path, it's essential to celebrate successes, overcome challenges, and seek out ongoing support and inspiration to stay motivated and committed to your goals.

Celebrating Successes on Atkins:

Whether you've just started Atkins or have been following the program for some time, it's important to acknowledge and celebrate your successes along the way. Celebrating milestones, big or small, can help boost your motivation and reinforce your commitment to the Atkins lifestyle.

One way to celebrate success on Atkins is by tracking your progress and setting achievable goals. Keep a journal or use a tracking app to monitor your weight loss, measurements, energy levels, and overall well-being. Celebrate reaching each milestone, whether it's losing a certain number of pounds, fitting into a smaller clothing size, or achieving a non-scale victory like improved sleep or increased energy.

Another way to celebrate success on Atkins is by treating yourself to rewards that align with your goals. Instead of using food as a reward, consider indulging in non-food rewards such as a massage, new workout gear, a spa day, or a fun activity that you enjoy. These rewards not only provide motivation but also reinforce positive behaviors and habits.

Furthermore, celebrate your successes by sharing them with others who support and encourage you on your journey. Whether it's friends, family, or fellow Atkins followers, sharing your achievements can help inspire others and create a sense of camaraderie and accountability.

Overcoming Challenges on Atkins:

While the Atkins diet offers numerous benefits, it's not without its challenges. From navigating social situations to dealing with cravings and setbacks, overcoming challenges is an integral part of the Atkins journey. Here are some strategies to help you overcome common challenges on Atkins:

1. **Social Situations**: Eating out, attending parties, and dining with friends and family can present challenges on Atkins. To navigate social situations successfully, plan ahead by reviewing menus, bringing Atkins-friendly snacks or dishes, and politely declining foods that don't align with your dietary goals. Give more thought to the company you keep than just the food.

2. **Cravings**: Cravings for high-carb foods can be a common challenge on Atkins, especially in the early stages. To combat cravings, focus on filling up on protein-rich foods, healthy fats, and fiber-rich vegetables to keep you feeling satisfied. Experiment with Atkins-approved recipes and snacks to satisfy your cravings without derailing your progress.

3. **Plateaus**: It's not uncommon to experience weight loss plateaus or stalls on Atkins, especially as your body adjusts to a new way of eating. If you

find yourself stuck in a plateau, reassess your dietary habits, increase your physical activity, and consider incorporating intermittent fasting or other strategies to kickstart your metabolism and break through the plateau.

4. **Mindset**: Adopting a positive mindset is crucial for overcoming challenges on Atkins. Instead of viewing setbacks as failures, reframe them as learning opportunities and opportunities for growth. Embrace self-compassion and acknowledge every accomplishment, no matter how tiny.

Resources for Ongoing Support and Inspiration on Atkins:

As you continue your Atkins journey, it's essential to seek out ongoing support and inspiration to help you stay motivated and committed to your goals. Fortunately, there are numerous resources available to support you every step of the way:

1. **Atkins Community**: Join the Atkins online community to connect with fellow followers, share success stories, ask questions, and find inspiration. The Atkins website offers forums, blogs, recipes, meal plans, and other valuable resources to support your journey.

2. **Social Media**: Follow Atkins on social media platforms like Facebook, Instagram, and Twitter for daily tips, recipes, success stories, and motivation. You can also join Atkins-related Facebook groups or Instagram communities to connect with like-minded individuals and share experiences.

3. **Atkins Books and Cookbooks**: Explore the wide range of Atkins books and cookbooks available, featuring expert advice, meal plans, recipes, and success stories. Whether you're looking for meal inspiration, nutritional guidance, or tips for success, Atkins books provide valuable resources to support your journey.

4. **Professional Support**: Consider seeking guidance from a registered dietitian or certified nutrition coach who specializes in low-carb diets like Atkins. A professional can provide personalized guidance, support, and accountability to help you reach your goals and overcome challenges.

5. **Podcasts and Webinars**: Listen to Atkins-related podcasts or attend webinars hosted by experts in the field for valuable insights, tips, and inspiration. These audio and video resources offer convenient ways to stay informed and motivated on your Atkins journey.

By tapping into these resources for ongoing support and inspiration, you can stay motivated, overcome challenges, and continue making progress on your Atkins journey toward better health and well-being. Remember that consistency, perseverance, and a positive mindset are key to long-term success on Atkins.

DAILY MEAL REMAKE

S/N	DAILY	MEAL	REMAKE
1.			